THE SILENT KILLER OF THE LIVER - NON-ALCOHOLIC FATTY LIVER DISEASE (NAFLD);

a piece of work designed to help you

learn how to take good care of

your liver by reversing, reducing, and preventing

non-alcoholic fatty liver disease (NAFLD).

by

I0446481

Dr. Robert J. Cardwell

TABLE OF CONTENTS

INTRODUCTION

In recent years, non-alcoholic fatty liver disease has drawn substantial attention and clinical research interest owing to its link with obesity, insulin resistance, metabolic syndrome, and cardiovascular illnesses. Non-alcoholic fatty liver disease (NAFLD) is a frequent and serious health issue that is on the increase globally. Its relationship with obesity, type 2 diabetes, and metabolic syndrome underscores the necessity of adopting a healthy lifestyle that combines regular exercise, a balanced diet, and weight control. Early identification and management are critical in limiting the development of NAFLD to more serious liver illnesses such as non-alcoholic steatohepatitis (NASH) and cirrhosis.

The Definition and Epidemiology (the study of the factors, prevalence, and distribution of health and illness in a specified population) of non-alcoholic fatty liver disease

NAFLD is characterized by the presence of hepatic steatosis, defined as fat accumulation surpassing 5% of the liver's weight, in the absence of any other recognized causes of liver disease. It is believed that NAFLD affects roughly 25% of the adult population worldwide, with greater incidence rates in Western nations. Also, it is increasingly becoming a prominent cause of liver-related morbidity and death, needing a fuller knowledge of its etiology, risk factors, and suitable therapeutic measures.

PATHOGENESIS:

The pathophysiology of NAFLD is complicated and includes a complex interaction of genetic, environmental, and metabolic factors. It is closely related to diseases such as obesity, type 2 diabetes mellitus, dyslipidemia, insulin resistance, and metabolic syndrome. Excessive accumulation of triglycerides in hepatocytes due to increased fatty acid uptake and de novo lipogenesis (a complex and highly regulated process in which carbohydrates from circulation are converted into fatty acids that are then used for synthesizing either triglycerides or other lipid molecules), coupled with impaired lipid metabolism and increased oxidative stress, resulting in hepatocellular injury, inflammation, and fibrosis. This finally leads to the progression of the illness and the development of more serious liver problems.

CLINICAL MANIFESTATIONS AND DIAGNOSIS:

In its early stages, NAFLD is generally asymptomatic and incidentally found on imaging exams conducted for other reasons. However, as the illness advances, some persons may have nonspecific symptoms such as weariness, malaise, and right upper quadrant stomach pain. Laboratory examinations may indicate increased liver enzymes (AST and ALT), however, they may not consistently correspond with the amount of liver damage. Diagnosis of NAFLD entails ruling out other liver illnesses (such as alcoholic liver disease and viral hepatitis) and confirming hepatic steatosis either using imaging methods (ultrasound, computed tomography, magnetic resonance imaging) or liver histology.

Suppose you are interested in the health and the general welfare of your liver. In that case, I urge that you acquire this book as it will enable you to learn further about how to reverse and finally eradicate the chronic impact of non-alcoholic fatty liver disease that kills quietly. Thus, join me in taking adequate care of your liver by clicking on the 'buy button' icon immediately.

CHAPTER 1

WHAT IS FATTY LIVER?

The liver is the largest organ within the body and is responsible for several vital processes that assist permit metabolism, immunity, digestion, detoxification, and vitamin storage. It is the only organ in the body capable of repairing after injury, yet numerous disorders may hurt it beyond the point of restoration. It is normal for the liver to have some fat. However, fatty liver or steatosis develops when 5-10% of the liver's weight is fat.

WHAT CAUSES FATTY LIVER?

Most persons with fatty liver do not have symptoms even as the condition worsens. This silent condition may develop into cirrhosis or liver cancer if left untreated.

WHAT IS THE MAIN CAUSE OF A FATTY LIVER?

The two primary kinds of fatty liver disease are nonalcoholic and alcoholic fatty liver disease.

NONALCOHOLIC FATTY LIVER DISEASE (NAFLD)

About 100 million individuals in the United States are believed to have nonalcoholic fatty liver disease. It happens when extra fat builds up in the liver cells unrelated to severe alcohol intake. NAFLD mainly affects those who are overweight and obese. Having diabetes, high cholesterol, or high triglycerides might also raise your chance of getting NAFLD. Rapid weight loss and bad eating habits may also contribute to this illness. The two kinds of NAFLD are simple fatty liver and nonalcoholic steatohepatitis (NASH).

ALCOHOLIC FATTY LIVER DISEASE (ALCOHOLIC STEATOHEPATITIS)

Each time you consume alcohol, some of your liver cells die. Prolonged alcohol usage over time might result in serious and irreversible liver damage. Alcoholic fatty liver disease is the initial stage of alcohol-related liver disease which may develop into alcoholic hepatitis and cirrhosis.

WHAT ARE THE SYMPTOMS OF FATTY LIVER?

Both kinds of fatty liver disease are silent illnesses with little or no symptoms. When symptoms emerge, a person may have stomach discomfort in the upper right side of the abdomen and occasionally exhaustion. Doctors may use blood testing, imaging studies, and occasionally, a biopsy to identify fatty liver disease.

Before we dig into more information connected to NAFLD, it is vital to grasp what alcoholic liver disease is.

ALCOHOLIC LIVER DISEASE

Alcohol-associated liver damage is caused by excessive consumption of alcohol. The liver's role is to break down alcohol. If you drink more than it can digest, it might get gravely injured. The steatotic (fatty) liver may arise in anybody who drinks a lot of alcohol. The graphic below will aid in a better understanding of the position and structural placement of the liver about other organs of the human body.

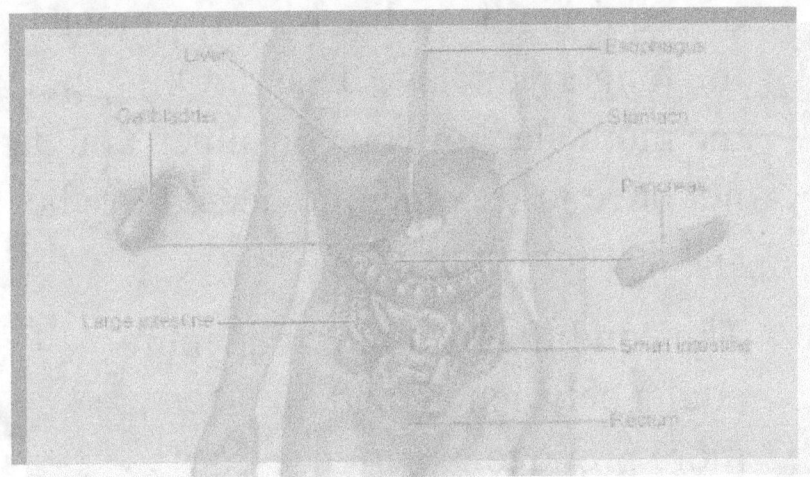

CAUSES OF ALCOHOLIC LIVER DISEASE

Alcoholic liver disease mainly happens after years of excessive drinking. Over time, scarring and cirrhosis might ensue. Cirrhosis is the last phase of alcoholic liver damage.

Alcoholic liver damage does not develop in all heavy drinkers. The odds of acquiring liver disease grow greater the longer you have been drinking and the more alcohol you consume. You do not have to become intoxicated for the sickness to happen.

The condition is more frequent in adults between 40 and 50. Men are more prone to experience this condition. However, women may get the condition with less exposure to alcohol than males. Some individuals may have a hereditary risk for the condition.

Long-term alcohol misuse may lead to serious damage termed alcoholic liver disease. Let's chat now about alcoholic liver illness. Alcoholic liver damage generally comes after years of drinking too much. The longer you've misused alcohol, and the more alcohol you've taken, the higher the probability you may get liver damage. Alcohol may induce swelling and inflammation in your liver, or something called hepatitis. Over time, this may progress to scarring and cirrhosis of the liver, which is the last phase of alcoholic liver disease. The damage induced by cirrhosis is sadly irreversible.

To establish whether you have alcoholic liver disease your doctor will usually test your blood, take a biopsy of the liver, and undertake a liver function test. It would help if you also underwent further tests to rule out other disorders causing your symptoms. Your symptoms may differ depending on the severity of your ailment. Usually, symptoms are worse following a recent period of excessive drinking. You may not even have symptoms until the illness is fairly advanced.

Generally, signs of alcoholic liver disease include stomach discomfort and soreness, dry mouth and increased thirst, weariness, jaundice (which is yellowing of the skin), lack of appetite, and nausea. Your skin may seem unnaturally dark or light. Your feet or hands may seem red. You may observe little, red, spider-like blood veins on your skin. You may have abnormal bleeding. Your stools can be dark, red, black, or tarry. You may have frequent nosebleeds or bleeding gums. You may vomit blood or something that looks like coffee grounds.

 Alcoholic liver disease also might harm your brain and nerve system. Symptoms include agitation, shifting mood, disorientation, discomfort, numbness, or a tingling feeling in your arms or legs. The most crucial element of rehab is to quit consuming alcohol. If you don't have liver cirrhosis yet, your liver can cure itself, that is, if you quit consuming alcohol.

You may need an alcohol recovery program or therapy to break free from alcohol. Vitamins, particularly B-complex vitamins, and folic acid, may help restore malnutrition. If cirrhosis develops, you will need to address the complications it might bring. It may potentially lead to requiring a liver transplant.

Having gained a decent understanding of what Alcoholic liver disease is, let's proceed with more information linked to non-alcoholic fatty liver disease.

CHAPTER 2

NON-ALCOHOLIC FATTY LIVER DISEASE (NAFLD)

Non-alcoholic fatty liver disease (NAFLD) as described previously is the name for a group of disorders caused by a build-up of fat in the liver. It's commonly noticed in folks who are overweight or obese.

Early-stage NAFLD does not normally cause any harm, but it may develop into major liver damage, including cirrhosis if it grows worse.

Having large amounts of fat in your liver is also related to an increased risk of major health concerns, such as diabetes, high blood pressure, and renal disease.

If you already have diabetes, NAFLD increases your probability of getting heart issues.

If discovered and controlled at an early stage, it's possible to halt NAFLD from growing worse and lower the amount of fat in your liver.

STAGES OF NON-ALCOHOLIC FATTY LIVER DISEASE (NAFLD)

NAFLD develops in 4 key phases.

Most individuals will only ever acquire the first stage, frequently without recognizing it.

In a tiny percentage of instances, it may develop and ultimately lead to liver damage if not recognized and addressed.

The primary phases of NAFLD are:

Simple fatty liver (steatosis) — a completely innocuous build-up of fat in the liver cells that may only be identified when testing is carried out for another cause

Non-alcoholic steatohepatitis (NASH) — a more severe variant of NAFLD, when the liver has become inflamed

Fibrosis - when recurrent inflammation forms scar tissue surrounding the liver and associated blood vessels, but the liver is still able to function properly.

Cirrhosis - the most severe stage, happening after years of inflammation, when the liver shrinks and becomes scarred and lumpy; this damage is permanent and may lead to liver failure (where your liver stops operating correctly) and liver cancer

It might take years for fibrosis or cirrhosis to develop. It's crucial to adopt lifestyle modifications to prevent the illness from growing worse.

HOW MUCH FATAL IS NON-ALCOHOLIC LIVER DISEASE?

The severity and possible mortality of NAFLD might vary significantly depending on the exact disease present.

The two primary kinds of NAFLD are non-alcoholic fatty liver (NAFL) and non-alcoholic steatohepatitis (NASH). NAFL normally does not cause major liver damage or proceed to late stages.

On the other side, NASH is a more severe variant of NAFLD, including inflammation and liver cell destruction. It may progress to fibrosis (scarring) of the liver, cirrhosis, and even liver failure. Cirrhosis is the most advanced stage and has an elevated chance of liver cancer as well.

The mortality of NAFLD relies on various variables, including the individual's general health, the existence of other illnesses (such as diabetes or obesity), the level of liver damage, and lifestyle adjustments. In general, the majority of persons with NAFLD will not develop serious consequences or mortality. However, a tiny number of persons with NASH may proceed to severe liver disease, necessitating liver transplantation or terminating in death.

Nonalcoholic steatohepatitis (NASH) is a severe type of nonalcoholic fatty liver disease (NAFLD), and it may proceed to cirrhosis and liver failure. The life expectancy for persons with NASH varies based on numerous variables, such as the course of the illness, the presence of other medical disorders, and the success of therapy.

NASH LIVER LIFE EXPECTANCY

On average, patients with NASH may have a life expectancy equivalent to that of the normal population if the condition is recognized early and handled successfully. However, in situations when NASH advances to extensive liver fibrosis or cirrhosis, the life expectancy might be considerably decreased. These patients may develop problems such as liver failure, portal hypertension, and hepatocellular carcinoma (liver cancer), which may further impair life expectancy.

It's crucial to note that lifestyle adjustments like as keeping a healthy weight, following a balanced diet, exercising frequently, controlling diabetes and cholesterol levels, and avoiding alcohol may help delay or prevent the advancement of NASH. Additionally, early identification and treatment of NASH might improve results and enhance life expectancy. It is important to speak with a healthcare practitioner for an accurate evaluation of individual prognosis and suitable therapy.

HOW COMMON IS FATTY LIVER?

The prevalence of nonalcoholic fatty liver disease (NAFLD) varies across locations and people. In the United States, NAFLD is a major problem and has become the most prevalent cause of chronic liver disease. It is believed that roughly 30% of individuals in the United States have NAFLD.

Globally, NAFLD is also a big health concern. It is believed that NAFLD affects roughly 25% of the worldwide population. The prevalence of NAFLD varies across nations, with certain areas having greater rates. It is more widespread in industrialized nations, especially in Western countries, where there is a larger incidence of obesity, sedentary lifestyles, and bad food habits.

The worldwide increase in the incidence of NAFLD is intimately connected to the growth in obesity, type 2 diabetes, metabolic syndrome, and other associated disorders. Additionally, changes in dietary patterns and lifestyle practices are contributing to the increased burden of NAFLD globally.

WHAT DOES A FATTY LIVER LOOK LIKE?

The image below shows what a healthy and sick liver looks like.

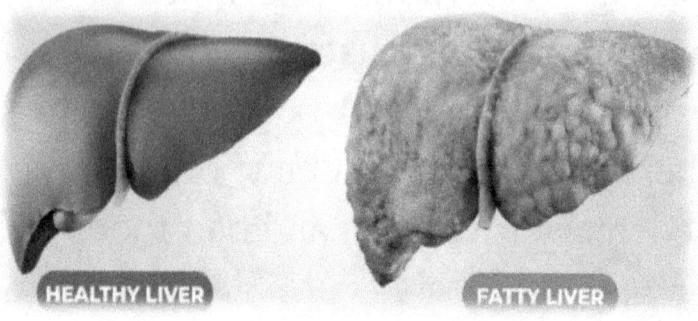

DOES FATTY LIVER CAUSE DIARRHEA?

Diarrhea is a disorder characterized by loose, watery bowel motions happening more often than normal. It may be caused by several circumstances, including infections, dietary changes, pharmaceutical side effects, and gastrointestinal issues. However, fatty liver disease itself is not considered a primary cause of diarrhea.

The reason for this is that fatty liver disease predominantly affects the liver, which plays a critical role in the metabolism of fat and the detoxification of numerous chemicals in the body. When the liver is damaged by excess fat deposition, it may lead to inflammation and scarring, which may result in hepatic dysfunction. However, the major function of the liver is not directly connected to the management of bowel motions or the digestive process.

Diarrhea is usually connected with illnesses that impact the intestines, such as infections, inflammatory bowel disease, or malabsorption problems. In some circumstances, the usual absorption and digestion of nutrients in the intestines are interrupted, resulting in abnormalities in bowel movements. Fatty liver disease, on the other hand, predominantly affects the liver and does not immediately damage the intestines or the process of digestion and absorption.

It's crucial to remember that although fatty liver disease may not directly cause diarrhea, it may contribute to overall digestive discomfort and may be connected with other symptoms that impact bowel movements, such as abdominal pain or bloating. If someone with fatty liver disease develops prolonged or severe diarrhea, it is essential to visit a healthcare practitioner to identify the underlying cause and give appropriate therapy

CHAPTER 3

MODERATE FATTY LIVER

Moderate fatty liver, also known as moderate hepatic steatosis, refers to a stage of fatty liver disease when there is a moderate buildup of fat in the liver cells. Fatty liver disease is divided into three stages: mild, moderate, and severe, depending on the level of fat accumulation and related liver damage.

In moderate fatty liver, the liver has a larger quantity of fat compared to the mild stage. The buildup of fat occurs inside the liver cells (hepatocytes) and may be observed by imaging methods such as ultrasound, computed tomography (CT) scan, or magnetic resonance imaging (MRI).

The existence of mild fatty liver might be a consequence of numerous reasons. The most prevalent cause is excessive alcohol intake, which leads to alcoholic fatty liver disease. Other factors include obesity, insulin resistance, metabolic syndrome, diabetes, high cholesterol, certain drugs, and fast weight reduction.

While moderate fatty liver is still considered a treatable disease, it implies a more substantial degree of fat buildup and may be accompanied by mild inflammation and liver cell damage. If left untreated or mismanaged, moderate fatty liver may proceed to severe fatty liver disease, also known as steatohepatitis, which includes inflammation and liver cell destruction. This may further develop into fibrosis, cirrhosis, and finally liver failure in extreme situations.

Management of moderate fatty liver focuses on treating the underlying causes and implementing lifestyle improvements to minimize fat buildup and enhance liver health. This may include:

1. Lifestyle changes: Adopting a balanced diet low in saturated and trans fats, increasing physical exercise, keeping a healthy weight, and avoiding excessive alcohol use are key measures in treating mild fatty liver.

2. Drugs: In certain circumstances, drugs may be administered to control underlying illnesses such as diabetes, high cholesterol, or metabolic syndrome, which may lead to fatty liver disease.

3. Regular monitoring: Individuals with mild fatty liver may be recommended to undertake periodic liver function tests and imaging scans to monitor the course of the condition and evaluate liver health.

4. Treatment of underlying problems: If fatty liver disease is connected with underlying disorders like diabetes or high cholesterol, controlling such conditions successfully will help improve fatty liver as well.

It's vital to remember that the therapy technique may differ based on the person and underlying issues. Therefore, it is suggested to visit a healthcare expert for a comprehensive diagnosis, assessment, and tailored treatment plan for mild fatty liver.

IS A FATTY LIVER HARMFUL?

While a fatty liver alone may not be harmful in the early stages, it may proceed to a more severe illness termed nonalcoholic steatohepatitis (NASH), which can be potentially deadly. NASH is characterized by inflammation and liver cell destruction in addition to the buildup of fat in the liver.

The inflammation and damage produced by NASH may lead to more major health concerns. NASH may proceed to cirrhosis, which is the advanced stage of liver scarring and can lead to liver failure. It may also raise the chance of getting liver cancer. NASH is currently considered one of the primary reasons for liver transplantation.

Moreover, fatty liver disease, including NASH, is related to an increased risk of cardiovascular illnesses, such as heart attacks and strokes. It is also strongly associated with obesity, type 2 diabetes, dyslipidemia (abnormal blood lipid levels), and metabolic syndrome, all of which may have major health repercussions.

Therefore, although a fatty liver may not be immediately harmful, it is vital to address the underlying causes, make lifestyle changes, and seek medical guidance to avoid the advancement of the condition and lower the related health risks.

ALKALINE PHOSPHATASE HIGH (MAJOR SYMPTOM)

Alkaline phosphatase (ALP) is an enzyme that is present in different tissues throughout the body, including the liver, bones, intestines, and kidneys. Elevated levels of ALP in blood tests may suggest liver and bone problems. In the context of fatty liver disease, elevated ALP levels are not regarded as a primary symptom, although they may be related to specific complications of the illness or other conditions.

In nonalcoholic fatty liver disease (NAFLD), the predominant symptom is the buildup of fat in the liver. NAFLD may be asymptomatic or may show nonspecific symptoms such as tiredness, minor stomach pain, or hepatomegaly (enlarged liver). However, these symptoms are not particular to fatty liver disease and may occur in several other illnesses as well.

Elevated ALP levels detected in blood tests are more usually related to other liver disorders such as primary biliary cholangitis, primary sclerosing cholangitis, or blockage of the bile ducts. These disorders may be present alongside or due to fatty liver disease.

It is crucial to note that diagnosing fatty liver disease often needs complete assessment, including a mix of medical history, physical examination, blood tests, imaging techniques (such as ultrasound, CT scan, or MRI), and occasionally a liver biopsy for confirmation. ALP levels alone are not adequate to establish a diagnosis of fatty liver disease, but they may give additional information when evaluated in the context of other liver function tests and clinical symptoms.

If you feel you have fatty liver disease or have high ALP levels, it is advisable to speak with a healthcare expert for thorough examination and assistance. They will be able to analyze your unique condition and make suitable advice and treatment alternatives based on the results.

CHAPTER 4

HOW TO REVERSE A FATTY LIVER

Reversing fatty liver disease entails adopting lifestyle improvements and treating the underlying causes of the problem. Here are some ways that may help:

1. Maintain a healthy weight: Losing extra weight is vital in controlling fatty liver disease. Gradual and consistent weight reduction with a balanced diet and regular exercise may help decrease liver fat and enhance liver function. Aim for a moderate weight reduction of 1-2 pounds each week.

2. Follow a healthy diet: Focus on a diet that is minimal in added sugars, processed carbs, and saturated fats. Instead, prioritize fruits, vegetables, whole grains, lean protein sources

(such as fish, chicken, and lentils), and healthy fats (such as avocados, nuts, and olive oil). Ensure an appropriate diet of important nutrients including vitamins E, C, and D. Avoid or minimize alcohol usage since it might cause liver damage.

3. Increase physical activity: Regular exercise may help burn extra fat, increase insulin sensitivity, and boost general health. Aim for at least 150 minutes of moderate-intensity aerobic activity each week, combined with strength training activities twice a week.

4. Manage underlying conditions: If you have related conditions like obesity, type 2 diabetes, or dyslipidemia, cooperate with your healthcare professional to manage and control these symptoms efficiently.

This may require drugs, dietary adjustments, and frequent monitoring.

5. Avoid hazardous substances: Minimize exposure to poisons and chemicals that may affect the liver. This includes avoiding excessive alcohol intake, smoking, and exposure to dangerous chemicals.

6. Seek medical advice: It is crucial to collaborate with your healthcare professional for thorough assessment, monitoring, and direction. They can analyze the severity of your fatty liver disease and give specific advice and treatment alternatives.

Remember, curing fatty liver disease requires time and effort. It is crucial to create permanent lifestyle adjustments and maintain a healthy habit in the long term. Regular follow-ups with your healthcare practitioner may assist in monitoring your progress and making any necessary modifications to your treatment plan.

THE ICD-10 CODE FOR NASH CIRRHOSIS

The ICD-10 code for NASH cirrhosis is K74.6. ICD-10 (International Classification of Illnesses, 10th Revision) is a medical coding system used by healthcare professionals to define and identify particular illnesses, medical conditions, and treatments. It enables standardization in paperwork, invoicing, and statistical analysis.

The designation K74.6 comes within the wider category of "Other and unspecified cirrhosis of the liver" (K74). Within this group, it especially reflects cirrhosis induced by nonalcoholic steatohepatitis (NASH).

This number is used to identify and monitor instances of NASH cirrhosis in medical records, for billing reasons, and statistical study of liver disease prevalence and treatment.

HEPATIC STEATOSIS TREATMENT

The therapy of hepatic steatosis, or fatty liver disease, focuses on lifestyle modifications and treating any underlying problems that may contribute to the illness. Here are some popular techniques for treatment:

1. Weight loss: If you are overweight or obese, decreasing weight is often a crucial component of therapy. Gradual and consistent weight reduction by diet adjustments and regular exercise may help decrease liver fat and enhance liver function. It is advisable to strive

for a moderate weight reduction of 1-2 pounds each week.

2. Diet modifications: Following a healthy and balanced diet helps control hepatic steatosis. This involves limiting intake of processed foods, sugary drinks, and saturated fats, and increasing consumption of fruits, vegetables, whole grains, lean proteins, and healthy fats. Limiting alcohol usage is crucial as well.

3. Regular exercise: Engaging in regular physical activity can increase insulin sensitivity, decrease liver fat, and enhance overall health. Aim for at least 30 minutes of moderate-intensity exercise most days of the week. Consult with a healthcare expert before beginning any workout regimen.

4. Management of underlying illnesses: If you have other medical disorders that

contribute to hepatic steatosis, such as diabetes, high cholesterol, or high blood pressure, it is crucial to address these conditions appropriately. This may require drugs, lifestyle adjustments, and frequent monitoring.

5. Avoidance of hepatotoxic chemicals: Certain drugs and substances may be detrimental to the liver. It is vital to prevent or reduce the use of hepatotoxic substances, such as excessive alcohol, certain medicines, and illegal narcotics, since these might cause hepatic steatosis.

6. Regular monitoring: Regular medical check-ups and monitoring of liver function via blood tests may assist in evaluating the development of the illness and the efficiency of therapy. Your healthcare practitioner may also offer imaging investigations, such as

ultrasonography or fibroScan, to examine liver function and the amount of liver damage.

It's vital to remember that the treatment technique may differ based on the severity of the condition and individual circumstances. It is essential to speak with a healthcare practitioner for individualized advice and help in controlling hepatic steatosis.

HOW LONG IT TAKES FOR FATTY LIVER DISEASE TO TURN INTO CIRRHOSIS

This illness is reversible and does not usually lead to more serious liver damage such as cirrhosis. However, in certain situations, if left untreated or inadequately managed, fatty liver disease may proceed to a more severe stage termed cirrhosis.

The development of fatty liver disease to cirrhosis varies from person to person and is affected by several variables such as individual susceptibility, lifestyle, genetics, and the existence of other underlying illnesses such as alcohol misuse, viral hepatitis, or metabolic abnormalities.

The timetable for fatty liver disease to proceed to cirrhosis is not well-defined and may vary from several years to decades. This process normally happens in three stages:

1. Steatosis (Simple fatty liver): In this early stage, the liver stores extra fat but has little to no inflammation or liver cell injury. Most persons with simple fatty liver do not suffer severe symptoms, and the illness may typically be found accidentally by

imaging studies or blood tests indicating raised liver enzymes. With adequate lifestyle adjustments, including weight reduction, dietary improvements, and exercise, simple fatty liver may be reversed and controlled well.

2. Non-alcoholic steatohepatitis (NASH): If left untreated, some patients with fatty liver disease may develop NASH, a more severe type marked by inflammation and liver cell damage. Over time, NASH may lead to the development of fibrosis, a process in which liver tissue is replaced by scar tissue. Fibrosis is a vital step toward the development of cirrhosis. The pace at which fibrosis occurs may vary greatly across people. While some may develop swiftly, others may stay stable for a lengthy time or even regress with

proper lifestyle modifications and medical therapies.3.

CIRRHOSIS: It's the advanced stage of liver disease marked by severe scarring and irreparable liver damage. At this stage, liver function is considerably reduced, and symptoms such as jaundice, ascites (fluid buildup in the abdomen), easy bruising, weariness, and cognitive impairment may arise. If not controlled or treated effectively, cirrhosis may progress to liver failure, liver cancer, or even death.

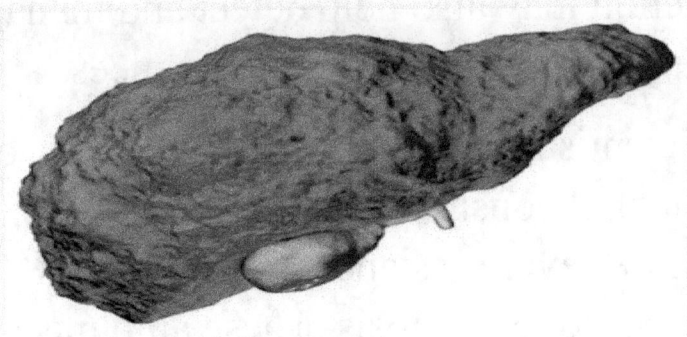

Cirrhotic liver

It is crucial to highlight that not all persons with fatty liver disease proceed to cirrhosis. By adopting a healthy lifestyle, including a balanced diet, frequent exercise, avoiding excessive alcohol use, managing obesity, and addressing underlying medical disorders, it is generally feasible to slow down or prevent the development of fatty liver disease to cirrhosis. Regular medical check-ups and early action may also help detect and manage any risk factors and consequences.

Scientists consider specific amounts of alcohol consumption to indicate how more severe instances of ALD may proceed to cirrhosis. These amounts are 40–80 grams (g) of ethanol per day for men and 20–40 g for females. If a person drinks these doses of alcohol regularly, their AFLD may proceed to cirrhosis in 10–12 years.

People with NAFLD may develop NASH and NAFLD-related cirrhosis over 3-6 years. However, a person's risk relies on several variables, including:

Diabetes

 Body mass

Hypertension

Menopause

Genetic factors

CHAPTER 5

WHAT CAUSES COMPLETE LIVER DAMAGE?

Cirrhosis is a disorder where the liver is permanently damaged and scarred. The scar tissue from cirrhosis replaces healthy liver tissue and inhibits blood flow. Cirrhosis might ultimately cause the liver to fail.

Symptoms People may have no symptoms until cirrhosis has destroyed their liver. Early signs may include Fatigue.

Weakness.

Poor appetite.

Weight loss without a clear reason

Nausea.

Vomiting.

Pain in the upper right side of the abdomen

Later symptoms may include Easy bleeding or bruising.

Sleep problems.

Mental symptoms such as Confusion.

Memory loss.

Difficulty thinking.

Personality changes.

Severely itching skin.

Darker urine color,

Jaundice, a yellow tinge to the whites of the eyes and skin edema, swelling in the lower legs, ankles, or feet ascites, an accumulation of fluid in the belly that produces bloating.

Cirrhosis may lead to liver failure and other problems.

Treatment

Doctors attempt to address the underlying cause of a person's cirrhosis to help prevent it from deteriorating or causing liver failure.

WHAT IS THE OUTLOOK FOR CIRRHOSIS?

The prognosis for a person's cirrhosis relies on its advancement. There are two phases of cirrhosis:

Compensated cirrhosis: People with compensated cirrhosis have no symptoms. The life expectancy for patients with this stage is roughly 12 years.

Decompensated cirrhosis: People with decompensated cirrhosis have one or more signs or consequences. They may require a liver transplant. The life expectancy for patients with this stage is roughly 2 years.

People may be able to turn cirrhosis from decompensated to compensate by treating the underlying cause.

Read more about the prospects for cirrhosis.

Food and beverages that help repair a fatty liver

Eating natural, unprocessed meals that provide complex carbs, fiber, and protein is a wonderful beginning point. These may give continuous energy and help a person feel full.

Some individuals opt to follow certain diet patterns, such as the Mediterranean diet. This diet is a particularly appropriate option for persons with NAFLD since it reduces processed food, added sugar, and saturated fatty acids.

Depending on the kind of fatty liver disease a person has, a dietitian may assist in building a tailored food plan that is suited to their preferences, symptoms, and health condition.

Some particular foods that may be especially useful for patients with fatty liver disease include:

Garlic

Garlic is a mainstay in many cuisines, and it may give advantages to those with fatty liver disease. A 2022 review indicated that garlic supplements had a beneficial influence on the metabolic profile of persons with NAFLD.

Omega-3 fatty acids

A 2020 assessment of existing evidence reveals that ingesting omega-3 fatty acids may reduce liver fat, high-density lipoprotein cholesterol levels, and BMI in persons with NAFLD.

Foods that are rich in omega-3 fatty acids include:

Salmon

Sardines

Walnuts

Flaxseed

Coffee

Drinking coffee is a morning habit for many individuals. However, it may give advantages beyond a surge of energy for those with fatty liver disease.

A 2020 meta-analysis indicated that frequent coffee drinking is strongly connected with a lower risk of liver fibrosis development in patients diagnosed with NAFLD.

Liver fibrosis develops when large quantities of scar tissue build up in the liver owing to recurrent or long-lasting damage or inflammation.

Another research from 2021 also indicated there is a possibly positive impact of coffee drinking on the severity of liver fibrosis in NAFLD patients.

Broccoli

Eating a range of whole vegetables is useful for persons with fatty liver disease, and broccoli is one vegetable that a person with fatty liver disease can consider having in their diet.

A 2022 animal research published in The Journal of Functional Foods discovered that broccoli helped the liver of mice with NAFLD break down lipids quicker, minimizing their build-up.

Researchers still need to perform more investigations involving people. However, early research on the influence of broccoli intake on the development of fatty liver disease appears encouraging.

Green tea

Using tea for therapeutic reasons is a tradition that stretches back thousands of years.

Green tea offers various antioxidants, such as catechin. Research shows that these antioxidants may help relieve the symptoms of fatty liver disease.

Walnuts

While all tree nuts are an excellent complement to any diet plan, walnuts are notably abundant in omega-3 fatty acids and may give advantages to patients with fatty liver disease.

Although additional research is required, a 2023 review in the journal Nutrients identified a substantial relationship between nut consumption and a lower incidence of NAFLD.

Soy or whey protein

A 2019 research in the journal Nutrients revealed that soy and whey protein decreased fat formation in the liver.

The findings of one trial in the review indicated that liver fat dropped by 20% in women with obesity who ate 60 grams (g) of whey protein per day for 4 weeks.

Soy protein includes antioxidants called isoflavones that help enhance insulin sensitivity and decrease fat in the body.

FOOD AND DRINKS TO AVOID

Adding nutritious foods to the diet is one method to control fatty liver disease. However, it is just as crucial for persons with this illness to avoid or restrict their consumption of certain other foods.

Sugar and added sugars

According to the AGA's Clinical Practice Update, persons with fatty liver disease, in particular NAFLD, should avoid or restrict added sugars. These may lead to elevated blood sugar levels and increased fat in the liver.

Manufacturers regularly add sugar to confectionery, ice cream, and sweetened beverages such as soda and fruit drinks. Added sugars also occur in packaged meals, baked products, and even store-bought coffee and tea.

Avoiding other sweets, such as fructose and corn syrup, may also help decrease fat in the liver.

Alcohol

Excessive alcohol intake is a prominent avoidable cause of mortality in the

United States. Alcohol affects the liver, leading to fatty liver disease and other disorders, such as cirrhosis.

A person with fatty liver disease should aim to minimize their alcohol consumption or eliminate it from their diet completely.

Here, read more about the short- and long-term impacts of alcohol.

Refined grains

Processed and refined grains are prevalent in white bread, white pasta, and white rice. Producers remove the fiber from these highly processed grains, which can raise blood sugar as the body breaks them down.

Several studies have shown that those hose who consumed fewer refined grains had a lower risk of metabolic syndrome, a group of risk factors that increase the likelihood of various health issues.

People may substitute refined grains with potatoes, lentils, whole wheat, and whole grain alternatives.

Fatty, fried, or salty meals

Too much fatty, fried, or salty food is likely to increase calorie intake and can lead to a person developing obesity, a common cause of fatty liver disease.

Adding additional spices and herbs to a meal is a terrific way to flavor meals without adding salt. People can also generally bake or steam items instead of frying them.

Meat

A saturated fat intake increases the amount of fat around organs, including the liver.

Beef, pork, and deli meats are all rich in saturated fats. The AGA recommended that a person with fatty liver disease attempt to avoid these foods as much as possible.

Lean meats, fish, tofu, or tempeh provide excellent replacements. However, wild, oily fish may be the best option, since it also supplies omega-3 fatty acids

CONCLUSION

Non-alcoholic fatty liver disease is a complicated, multifaceted disorder with substantial consequences for world health. Its increased frequency and relationship with metabolic illnesses demand a full knowledge of its etiology, diagnosis, and therapy. Early detection, lifestyle adjustments, and effective treatment techniques are critical in reversing or preventing the course of NAFLD, thereby decreasing the burden of liver-related morbidities and mortality.

Further research and clinical investigations are necessary to discover innovative treatment targets and approaches in the realm of NAFLD management.

Non-alcoholic fatty liver disease (NAFLD) is a serious and developing issue globally. It is intimately connected with obesity, diabetes, and other metabolic problems. The progressive nature of NAFLD, from basic steatosis to more severe diseases like NASH and cirrhosis, underscores the significance of early identification and care. Lifestyle adjustments, including adopting a balanced diet, increasing physical exercise, and keeping a healthy weight, are crucial in the treatment and prevention of NAFLD.

Additionally, treating underlying medical issues, such as diabetes and excessive cholesterol, may greatly enhance liver health. Regular monitoring and follow-up, combined with competent medical assistance, are critical in controlling the condition and decreasing the risk of complications. Through a multimodal strategy, NAFLD may be successfully controlled, and the risk of development to severe liver disease can be decreased. Efforts should also be made to improve knowledge of the condition, its risk factors, and the necessity of early identification and care. By following these techniques, we can reduce the growing incidence of

NAFLD and enhance the overall health and well-being of persons impacted by this silent epidemic.

www.ingramcontent.com/pod-product-compliance
Lightning Source LLC
Chambersburg PA
CBHW062252290526
45794CB00006B/2510